Get Fit For Life
Virgin Fitness Tips

By Cathy Wilson

Copyright © 2014

Income Disclaimer

This book contains business strategies, marketing methods and other business advice that, regardless of my own results and experience, may not produce the same results (or any results) for you. I make absolutely no guarantee, expressed or implied, that by following the advice below you will make any money or improve current profits, as there are several factors and variables that come into play regarding any given business.

Primarily, results will depend on the nature of the product or business model, the conditions of the marketplace, the experience of the individual, and situations and elements that are beyond your control. As with any business endeavor, you assume all risk related to investment and money based on your own discretion and at your own potential expense.

Liability Disclaimer

By reading this book, you assume all risks associated with using the advice given below, with a full understanding that you, solely, are responsible for anything that may occur as a result of putting this information into action in any way, and regardless of your interpretation of the advice.

You further agree that our company cannot be held responsible in any way for the success or failure of your business as a result of the information presented in this book. It is your responsibility to conduct your own due diligence regarding the safe and successful operation of your business if you intend to apply any of our information in any way to your business operations.

Terms of Use

You are given a non-transferable, "personal use" license to this book. You cannot distribute it or share it with other individuals.

Also, there are no resale rights or private label rights granted when purchasing this book. In other words, it's for your own personal use only.

Get Fit For Life
Virgin Fitness Tips

By Cathy Wilson

Table of Contents

Introduction

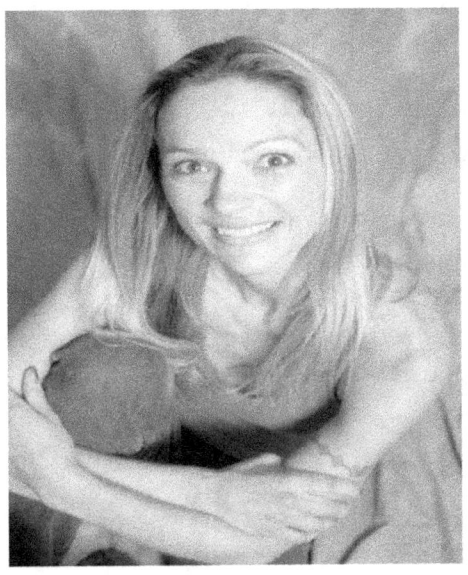

Get Fit For Life - Virgin Fitness Tips is all about gaining expert knowledge in health and wellness that's simplistic, logical, practical, and **FUN!**

I will use my deep fitness training knowledge to SHOW you, step-by-step, how to get fit long-term.

FACT - There's always something to improve, when getting your mind and body healthy.

An open mind is a beautiful thing.

This introductory book focuses on the importance of keeping the body physically active. It's about finding the exercise regimen that works with your preferences and tolerances, ability, and lifestyle; one that **WILL** stick for life.

The number one factor in exercise plan failure, according to *Shape* magazine, is not having a plan.

I not only help you create your fitness plan, but I also help you understand it.

Your regimen needs to be created, it's not going to magically appear. You've gotta *want* it!

According to *The American Heart Association*, regular exercise promotes weight reduction, reduces blood pressure, lowers LDL or *bad* cholesterol, and raises HDL or *good* cholesterol.

It all comes down to choice. Figuring out what type of exercising is effective for you, and focusing on it. You are important, and so is your good health. I give you the knowledge required to make better exercise decisions for you, steering you toward some easy long-term weight loss, and a permanent smile in the process.

If you gain just one piece of useful information to make YOU a better YOU, then I'm a very happy girl.

The golden ticket?

To make your new healthy choices habit, so they become your new *normal,* rather than a moment in time, that gets tossed aside for comfort and familiarity. Just think fad diets and crazy exercise programs, and you've got it. Sorry if I just stirred up some nightmares!

I'll give you the knowledge and practicality, to set yourself up for success, and support you throughout. One manageable step at a time, you **WILL** get you to the finish line with a smile. In better shape than yesterday.

Mind over matter. Never forget that!

Exercise Benefits

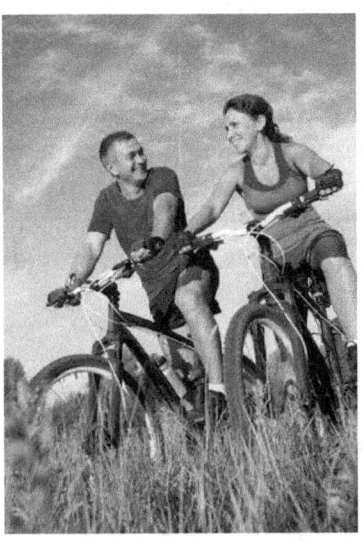

You're exercising when you go for a run, play an intense bump and grind basketball game, or just hike it up the stairs fast. It's that feeling of having to breathe deeper and longer, providing more oxygen to your heart, lungs, and internal systems, that are actually doing the work.

It's where your cardiovascular and muscles are in action. Working your lungs intensely and regularly, increases your cardiovascular capacity, helps build lean muscle strength for better overall fitness, and triggers a euphoric endorphin release, which feels much like the temporary energetic high a drug user feels, except it's legal, and a fantabulous addiction!

On the flip side, choosing to never challenge your body only leaves you weak and alone, creaky and cracky, starving off bothersome aches and pains forever, or until serious free radicals invade your internal system, and poison you with disease.

Exercise is your CONTROLLABLE PREVENTATIVE measure to fight disease, both physical and mental.

What is Cardiovascular specifically? Cardiovascular relates to the blood vessels and heart functioning, inclusive of veins and arteries. It's when you're participating in an exercise like running, increasing your heart rate, and forcing higher oxygen intake, while providing increased energy to perform.

Dynamic yoga, cycling, skating, rollerblading, circuits, swimming, and fast walking, are great examples of cardiovascular exercise.

When aerobic activity is applied to exercise, it's referred to as cardiovascular exercise. A key factor in weight loss, or conditioning training for athletes, for instance.

What is Muscle building? When you utilize muscles during exercise, you're building muscle. In short, by weight training muscles, you'll bulk up your muscle cells, helping your body burn more calories overall.

This also triggers a metabolic increase, cuz muscle burns more calories than fat on a level playing field. Muscle cells are also physically smaller than fat cells, appearing more compact and less jiggly than fat.

*FIT ALERT! Contrary to our programming from days past, women don't need to be afraid they'll look like a muscle **Hulkster** by weight training. Experts agree, this isn't true. A woman's body wasn't made with muscles cells that **normally** grow gynormous, like a man's.*

Women don't have the hormonal makeup, or the physical ability to get huge. Now, if you're fooling around with hormones, specifically growth hormones, under the guidance of a trainer and doctor, you can force your body to build more muscle than the average woman would. But these women have a specific focus, and are the exception to the rules. The best thing you can do for your physical body ladies, is to start pumping iron!

Add muscle building or strength training to your cardiovascular exercise, and you're going to build your body strong, running effectively head to toe. You'll increase your metabolism to blast fat faster, leaving you lookin' smoking hot, and feeling fantastico!

My thoughts . . .

You can't have one without the other. If you want the maximum benefits from exercising, you've gotta get your heart pumping, and muscles working hard with regular aerobic exercise, and muscle building strategies.

Starting off with at least 30 minutes of cardio three to four days a week, and two to three days of muscle building, for twenty minutes each time, should do the trick. It's a solid platform from which to build.

Don't try and be perfect. Just get your feet wet. Then you can set your parameters higher.

Did you know fitness professionals agree you need thirty to sixty minutes of exercise EVERY day for optimal health?

It's true, and let me tell you why.

History of Exercise

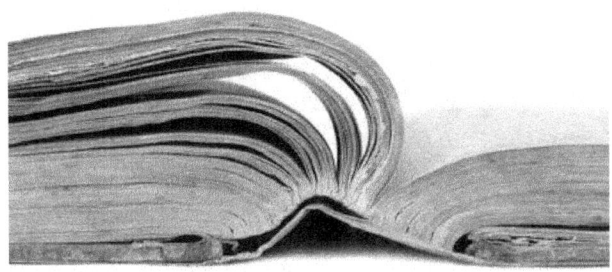

Exercise has been around since the beginning of time. In ancient days, people were naturally muscular and strong, because physical was their life. *Fittest of the fittest* was their reality.

These people relied on body strength and elite physical stamina for food, shelter, clothes, and survival, not like people today, where we can literally survive without getting out of bed.

Everything is automatic, pre-packaged, and preserved to death; a poison of convenience. It's the ultimate cost of progress.

People in the olden days had a full day of diverse exercise every time they wanted to eat. When lucky, they had a horse to hop on, grabbed their bow and arrow, or spear, and headed off miles into the bush to hunt game.

If their tracking skills were bang on, a tasty antelope or gazelle would be dinner. Ancient man would skillfully track and chase the game down, kill it, and drag it back to camp.

But they weren't done yet!

Usually the women got the skinning and cleaning job. While the men gathered firewood, and anything else required for the feast. Some days, the hunters might get lucky and catch a catnap, while the women cooked the long awaited feast.

Their basic needs remained constant. Each day was much the same, a fight for survival.

Hundreds of years ago, people didn't have to consciously think about exercising physically, mentally, or emotionally. They had no choice. Ancient people were stimulated mentally and emotionally, with all the dangers of the chase.

Wouldn't you be?

Their problem was opposite to modern day society, rarely getting the mental and physical rest necessary for optimal function.

We don't need the physical shut-down time like our ancestors. And when it comes to the mental, we create a gynormous amount of stress, often overwhelming, and do everything but deal with it.

So why do we need exercise?

Lack of exercise in our society today is self-created. By choosing to disassociate with the basic natural elements of human survival, we get lazy, and stress our health. Add lack of caloric burn through exercise, to programming ourselves to overeat all the wrong foods, and we've created a deadly combination.

Fatness, illness, and disease manifest, with preventable suffering, and eventual death to follow.

Weepy sad, but true.

NEWSFLASH! Your body was designed to require set amounts of lean protein, complex carbohydrates, good fats, various vitamins and minerals, and regular exercise; cardiovascular, weight lifting, strength training, toning, and stretching exercise ROUTINELY.

Depriving your body screws it up. Sorry, there's no *nice* way to say it.

If you want the opportunity to live a long, happy, healthy, productive, and fully mobile life, you'd better get crackin to improve your cardio, and muscular capacity.

You can choose to sit on your butt eating Twinkies, watching life pass you by, while letting the natural factors of aging, slowly take your physical ability to move without pain away, or worse.

Or, you can stand up and fight.

Make a commitment to find time to exercise, and program your mind to enjoy it every day. Time will pass you by regardless. It's up to you to take action for your good health.

How do you program your mind to enjoy exercise?

*Find exercise you enjoy
*Literally tell yourself you're enjoying it
*Look consciously for the positives in exercise
*Focus on getting results, so when you do, this inspires you naturally to want more

VIP - According to *Natural News and Scientific Discoveries,* personal development expert, *Noah St. John,* states positive affirmation is just the start of creating new healthy habits. By reminding yourself positively about your new exercise regimen, you'll begin to believe it.

Continue positively reminding yourself, and this belief grows strong, removing doubt and solidifying your belief, and new fantabulous habit.

I don't want to hear excuses. Experts agree, exercising of any sort benefits **EVERY** single being, health issues or not. Age does not factor in. Because whether you are 25 or 80, you can create an exercise plan that works for you.

The pros of exercising trumps all. Even if you've never worked up a sweat your entire life.

No excuses!

The proof is in the pudding. Get your heart rate pumping for even a few minutes, and you'll feel spectacular! A psychosomatic boost extraordinaire.

Further in **Get Fit for Life**, we'll look into the emotional, mental, and physical benefits of exercise in a broad scope, starting with exercise basics, your body, and thinking. Then we'll investigate how to prepare yourself for physical exercise. We'll look into some exercise lingo, workout ideas, and even some exercise equipment you may see fit to purchase, for your quest of getting strong, fit, and healthy.

FITNESS ALERT! Did you know, you were born with a set number of muscle and fat cells? So when you lose weight, you don't lose fat cells. They shrink when you send fat packing. By lifting weights, eating plenty of protein, and gaining muscle, new muscle cells aren't created either.

You're just strengthening ones you already have.

My thoughts. . .

There are gynormous benefits to exercising, and there's really no excuse not to. Exercise is fantastic for your mind and body.

For a bonus?

*There's nothing better than the natural feel **good feeling** after sweating up a storm. That satiating sense of energetic well-being, is like no other!*

Basic Benefits of Exercise

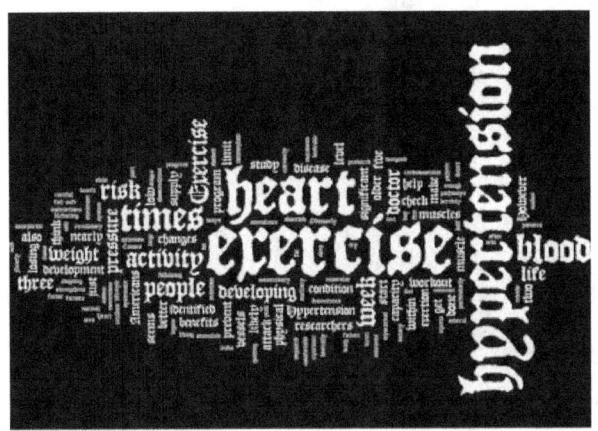

You should be proud deciding to bring the physical back into your every day. Change is never easy, adding the crazy busy life schedule most of us experience, makes finding the time to exercise a serious, but worthwhile challenge.

Here's a list of the basic benefits of exercise in a nutshell.

MENTAL

-Better mood (natural endorphins)
-Increased self-esteem
-Better mood
-Higher feeling of energy
-Lowers symptoms of anxiety and depression
-Better confidence

-Increased sense of pride
-Better able to deal with stress
-Improved reasoning in stressful situations
-Feel better about your looks
-Feel better about others perceptions of you
-Improved self-esteem

PHYSICAL/HEALTH

-Helps prevent annoying conditions and disease
-Lowers blood pressure
-Decreases the risk of heart disease, stroke, and other serious ailments
-Lowers the risk of numerous cancers, diabetes, and osteoporosis
-Strengthens muscles, bones, and supporting ligaments - preventing falls, and injuries
-Faster injury recovery time
-Tones and strengthens the body
-Weight loss
-Improvement in agility and mobility
-Less aches and pains
-Increases tolerance to pain
-Increases cardiovascular capacity
-Improves muscle endurance
-Lowers cholesterol levels
-Improves social benefits
-Improves circulatory function
-Improves skin, nails, and hair
-Aids in skin elasticity
-Decreases risk of back problems

Your health is important, and the above should be enough to convince you any exercising is good exercising.

Mentality - Anything is better than nothing

Now you know some benefits of sweating up a storm. Your next quest is to figure out exercise preferences, and timing. If you prefer group aerobics, then do it! Don't be afraid to experiment.

Time to figure out what works for you!

Aging is another inevitable fact of life.

Aging is the process in which your body naturally breaks down with time, an aspect of life we all share. You can choose to just accept the fact your muscles are going to break down, energy levels will start depleting, bones will weaken, and your skin will start to lose its vibrancy.

Or, you can choose to fight the aging process, and live a more fulfilling, longer healthier life.

Getting yourself into shape by exercising on a regular basis, is a tool to improve your looks, gain strength, and scare off disease, leaving you feeling better about yourself, and life as a whole.

This process of getting fit is going to take patience, time, and perseverance. One step at a time. One foot in front of the other. Always looking to make better decisions, without being too hard on yourself when you take a step backwards.

You're only human, right?

Physical exercise will better your health; mind, body, and soul, giving you the opportunity to live a longer, healthier, and more vibrantly fulfilling life, than you would otherwise, opening doors of opportunity that might otherwise remain shut.

That should be plenty to make you smile.

Be Prepared

*Stop and figure out what your fitness level is . . .

Before you decide to take on a new fitness routine; whether it's hiking, biking, aerobics, yoga, Pilates, boot camp training, or a gym circuit; it's important you take a step back and measure your fitness level and knowledge.

If you don't, frustration sets in because you're tackling a mountain made for experts, not beginners. Worse yet, you'll enter a level too high, and get seriously injured, neither of which helps your head or body reach your fitness goals.

A few factors to consider before you set your new fitness strategies extraordinaire:

***Age** - Sure, exercising was a whole lot easier in your teens. There weren't any aches and pains to worry about, and your attitude left you afraid of nothing. Invincible comes to mind!

Well, times have changed, you're getting older, and it's important to consider your wants and expectations logically. I'm not going to tell you there's any particular exercise routine you can't do. But I caution you to be sensible in training.

For instance, if you're enjoying your golden years, while battling osteoporosis, you may want to steer clear of rollerblading, particularly if you've never been on skates before.

That's a sensible move.

Football is another exercise option that was awesome when you were twenty. But do you really want to sacrifice your body to get into shape, now that you're fifty, with two young children? Probably not.

Just promise me you'll think before you *eeny-meeny-miney-moe* your exercise program, to build your body super sexy strong!

*Medical Conditions - VIP - For safety, be sure you run any new exercise desires by your medical provider PRIOR to starting. Don't you dare start something and hurt yourself, only to discover a few weeks later from your doctor pal, you shouldn't have been doing downward dogs in the first place!

Be smart and check first, just to be sure.

*Preferences and Tolerances - You know what tickles your fancy when it comes to exercising. If you can't stand the thought of exercising in a gym, then don't buy a gym membership. Instead, you could join a cycling group, or maybe try an outdoor boot camp.

If you get happy with the idea of working out with other people. Make sure you test the waters with some sort of group exercise class. Perhaps you want to try kickboxing, aqua-aerobics, or a yoga class. The key is to acknowledge likes and dislikes, and set yourself up for success.

*Commitment - Getting into better physical shape is going to require a commitment.

NEWSFLASH! - You lose if you only exercise for a few weeks and quit.

Making a habit of getting physically fit takes time, commitment, consistency, and patience. Give yourself a chance to get used to your new routine. If you do, you'll be surprised how much you learn to look forward to it.

The rule of thumb with experts is, 6-8 weeks minimum, before you'll start to get comfortable. That's according to fitness professionals at **shape**.com

Stick it out, cuz the rewards are priceless!

*Don't Quit - If you're just learning the ropes in great fitness, and find yourself frustrated or bored, don't quit! The only way this isn't going to work, is if you walk away.

It's better just to try something new, if you're frustrated with your program.

Maybe the cycling wasn't working for you? That's okay. Why not try getting a personal trainer, or testing out the pool? Keep trying until you find the exercise niches that you really enjoy, ones you can envision doing for the rest of your life.

That's what fitness is all about. It's a change for the better that sticks for the long run, simply because you deserve to be healthy and happy, and live a long and productive life.

*Set Reasonable Expectations - Sure it's great to jump right into your exercise regimen. But if you overdo it, you're opening the door to fail. Many fitness beginners make the mistake of trying to do too much too soon. They're pumped and hit the gym every single day for a few hours, thinking they can keep this pace up. When they don't, negativity sets in, and quitting becomes reality.

The solution?

Slow and steady wins the race. Take your time easing into fitness. Start with 2-3 days a week, and work your way up. Consider the big picture; your schedule, and the longer term. By making sure you set reasonable expectations, you're one step closer to reaching each one of your fitness goals.

There's something really important I want to mention, just to make sure you've got the correct information. There isn't a doctor or health and wellness specialist on the planet, that's going to tell you exercise is *bad* for you, regardless of your medical health status or age.

Fact is, the benefits of exercising outweigh the risks or negative effects, if there are any, which is great news for everyone.

This doesn't mean there aren't limitations for people with serious medical conditions, because there will be. But with a little bit of effort, there's fantabulous exercise out there for everyone. A positive health move that only creates better!

Walking around the block, or even lifting soup cans for weights is better than nothing!

Make sure when you start your new exercise routine, you begin slowly. Sure, you may be really excited to get going, and that's great. But trust me on this one. Give your body a chance to adjust, reducing the risk of injury.

Getting sidelined for a few months won't help when you're focused on finishing the race.

Fitness Alert - *Did you know the best way to keep your energy levels up, especially when working out, is to eat smaller meals regularly? By eating five or six mini-meals throughout the day, instead of two or three larger ones, you're going to provide your body with the constant energy it requires to run efficiently. If you skip meals, or only have a couple meals a day, your blood sugar levels are going to ride a roller coaster.*

This delivers energy highs and lows sporadically throughout the day, stressing your mood. Choosing smaller healthy food choices every two to three hours during the day, will give you everything required, to keep your energy levels sky high for good.

My thoughts....

It's very important not to jump into a new exercise regime, without thinking and planning. Zone in on making the best choices for you, preferably ones that get results fast, and that you enjoy enough to stick with.

Where there's a will, there's a way. Just take it one step at a time. Consciously look for the positive, and most importantly **BELIEVE!**

Exercise Lingo

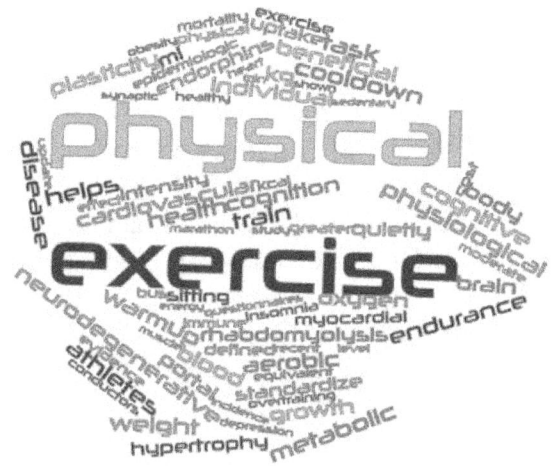

Unless you've got a fitness background, some of the lingo associated with getting fit really is quite confusing. By explaining some of the basic exercise talk, you'll have the firepower to make smarter workout decisions. *Mayo Clinic* states, it's important to become familiar with exercise terminology, to better apply effective strategies to get your body into shape faster.

*Preferences and Tolerances - This reflects owning up to and accepting what you really want, gearing your new exercise program towards what you enjoy, which increases your odds at succeeding.

For example, if you really don't like an exercise, don't do it! Simply make adjustments around it.

Perhaps you don't like lunges, or have bad knees. So either do half squats or 1/4 lunges instead. If you're uncertain, don't hesitate to ask a personal trainer. Better safe than sorry always.

*Practicality - If you live an hour away from the nearest gym, you have to decide if you're really going to drive all that way for a workout, after a long twelve hour shift?

Find a class closer to your work, or perhaps invest in some exercise equipment to get your heart pumpin' at home. There's no use committing to exercising, if you knowingly set yourself up to flunk.

Think smart and act smarter!

*Reps or Repetitions - Reps are a common term used to describe the number of times you repeat an exercise in one bout. Many people do ten reps of a particular weight in each set, which I'll explain next.

*Sets - Sets are groups of reps. For example, it's common to complete three sets of ten reps when executing biceps curls. This means you're going to do ten biceps curls in a row, and repeat this three times, with a short rest after every ten reps. I understand this can be a little confusing initially. It won't take you long to get comfortable after you get a few sets in.

*Rhythm - With exercising, this refers to the pace you're executing at. If you're doing squats, your rhythm may be in speed or count, maybe executing three faster squats, with a one count down, and one count up. Then next time, may be six squats, with a three count down, and two count up. This keeps your mind and muscles guessing, maximizing results.

*Weights - Weights are what you lift to work your muscles. In the gym, you'll find weight machines, barbells, medicine balls, and often kettle bells. The latter are just round weights with a handle, making them easier to grip and maneuver.

Weight training is used specifically for muscle building, helping you gain strength, burn calories more efficiently, increase metabolism, and blast pesky fat.

Fitness Alert - Did you know that muscle weighs more than fat? A muscular body is going to burn more calories than a fatty body of the similar dimension, which hammers home the fact, muscle building is flat-line critical for a healthy, fit, lean, and energetic body and mind.

*Muscle Building - A muscle is actually layers upon layers of muscle tissue, according to Livescience. About 40% of your body is muscle, and they're categorized as smooth, cardiac, and skeletal.

When building muscle, you isolate a set muscle, and work it specifically. Building muscle requires protein. When building lean muscle, you need 2-3 servings each day, simply because your body can't produce protein, nor does it store it. And if you don't have protein available to use, your body breaks down your muscles for energy.

Talk about defeating the purpose of sweating buckets to create sexy lean muscle!

EAT YOUR LEAN PROTEIN!

*Cardiovascular Activity - This activity exerts energy to increase heart rate, working hard to pump more oxygen and vital nutrients to your organs and bodily systems through your bloodstream.

It's also called aerobic exercise.

Aerobic refers to *living in air,* reflective of providing enough oxygen when your body is exercising.

Examples of cardiovascular activity are:

-Running
-Biking
-Hiking
-Swimming
-Aerobics class
-Kickboxing class
-Fast walking
-Treadmill
-Cross-Training
-Skating
-Circuits
-Tennis
-Soccer
-Cross country skiing

*Interval Training - This refers to alternating bouts of high level physical activity with lower level activity. It can mean running for three minutes, walking for one, and repeating. Or alternating between weights and cardiovascular activity, intensity, and duration. With interval training, you burn the maximum amount of energy, in the shortest amount of time, while utilizing diversity.

Just think circuit training here.

*Maximum Heart Rate - Is the maximum pace your heart should reach, according to age and genetics. This is a safety measure when exercising, to ensure you don't surpass your limitations.

It's just a guideline, and there are always exceptions to the rules.

Knowing where your maximum heart rate falls, allows for increased effectiveness.

*Resting Heart Rate - Is the rate your heart beats at rest. Technically, it's before you even move a muscle in the morning, even before getting your butt out of bed.

The lower your resting heart rate, the better shape you're in.

A fantabulous way to measure fitness progress.

*Heart Rate - Is essentially the number of times your heart beats per minute (bpm), at any given time. For instance, your heart rate's higher when adrenaline is pumping, and lower when you're chillin' for a snooze.

Fitness Alert - Many Get Fit for Life candidates, are worried about getting their heart rate too high. There are some pieces of cardio equipment, equipped with devices to calculate your heart rate. The purpose is to ensure you're in your safe zone. I would proceed with caution, because there have been numerous reports stating these readings are inaccurate. In fact, I have tested them on numerous occasions, and found them to be 20 or 30 beats off at times.

If you are in doubt, just opt for the talk test. When exercising, you should be able to talk, or hold a conversation with someone, without difficulty, unless you are in a specific training program. If you can't talk while training, you better slow it down.

*Stretching - Stretching isn't reaching your arms over your head for five seconds, rotating your arms around once or twice, and reaching down to the ground for another five seconds!

Proper stretching takes at least ten minutes, and for good reason. You're trying to warm your muscles up to workout out. You want them warm and *loose*, so you'll avoid injury even before you begin.

On that note, you should stretch before and after every workout session.

Stretching is physical exercise, where you choose a specific muscle group, tendon, or ligament, to isolate and stretch, or flex, in order to increase mobility.

Just picture your muscle as an elastic band. If you want it to stretch further, you need to gently stretch it further bit by bit. Stretching should always be slow and controlled, never bouncy or jerky, and it shouldn't hurt.

Each gentle stretch should be held for thirty seconds to a minute, and repeated.

*Forced Reps – This method of strength training is often used in body building, not something you'll be trying right now, but something to tuck away for future use.

Basically, it's when your body has reached muscle failure when lifting weights, where physically, you can't do any more reps. Of course, you need a spotter for this.

Instead of stopping when tired, you force yourself to do a few more, even though all your muscle fibers are telling you to stop. This shocks your system, ordering your body to stimulate more growth, because you're now using muscle fibers that are rarely, if ever, used.

This helps the biggest body builders get gynormous. Forced rep training is best done sporadically.

*Cool Down - This is where you slowly bring your heart rate down to your usual resting rate after exercising. So if you just finished an aerobics class, you'll spend about ten minutes slowing the pace down to a nice walk. Then do some gentle stretching, until you're completely cooled down.

*Warm Up - We touched on this a little already. Any time you exercise, you've gotta make habit of warming up! It's how you communicate to your body and mind, you're ready to train.

You might start with jumping jacks and a light jog to get your blood flowing. In your warm-up, you should include at least ten minutes of gentle stretching. This loosens your muscles and tendons, decreasing the risk of injury.

*Rest - This isn't referring to taking a nap. A rest or break in exercise, refers to a stop between sets while lifting weights, or a short break between exercises. It can also mean taking a break when training specific muscle groups.

For example, you don't want to work your back muscles two days in a row. Most people alternate muscle groups.

Rest can also refer to a break in training for your body to recharge and build muscle. This is especially important when training hard, and lifting heavy weights. If you don't rest adequately, you aren't going to get stronger or bigger.

*Supersets - These are another way to shock your system into giving you results, when executing strength training exercises. Typically, it's where you do two different exercises in a row, with no rest in between, followed by a cardio activity.

The idea is to alternate between muscle building and cardio exercises, and keep your heart rate up continuously. This method is fast and effective, a great way to break through those inevitable plateaus, where you just aren't getting results.

*Upper Body - These are all the muscle groups above your waist. Your arms, shoulders, back, and chest to start. Most people strength train their upper body specifically, one or two days a week, with a rest in between.

*Lower Body - Are all the muscle groups below the waist, your legs and buttocks. The same sort of training regimen applies as your upper body.

*Core - Your core is a group of muscles that help to stabilize, and move your different body segments. Think of it as the connecting factor between your upper and lower body.

The groups of muscles in your core are, your abdominals, hips, and back. Having a strong core is important in preventing, or minimizing back pain.

*Diversity - In exercising, this refers to changing things up. The more you diversify your workouts, the greater the results. By getting your head and body thinking, you'll force maximum effectiveness in your training.

In other words, you won't be able to coast on autopilot through your routine without thinking. You'll have to consciously focus on what you're doing with each exercise, which requires attention and concentration, maximizing your results, and minimizing the time spent getting there.

A boot camp training session is a fantastic example, cuz you combine a diverse range of high intensity interval training exercises, at your own pace, that are never the same twice.

Always changing is fantistico when it comes to fitness.

Fitness Alert - If I had to choose one activity to challenge all levels of fitness, it would be group boot camp sessions. These interval training sessions occur in a positive group atmosphere, driven by the energy in the room, and the abilities of the person next to you.

These sessions are set up to challenge you to beat your personal best EVERY time. Everyone is in the same boat, which is a motivator. These sessions combine a diverse range of cardio and muscle building exercises that can easily be modified personally, and still be effective.

For example, if you have bad knees, you don't have to do the squat station. Instead, you can do ab work, or pushups. And the instructors are always pushing and encouraging everyone to do better.

A fantabulous route to get results fast, regardless of your fitness level.

My Thoughts . . .

It's very important to understand some of the basic terms of fitness before applying. It may be a little intimidating to start. But I promise you, it won't be long before you're used to most of the lingo, and applying your newfound knowledge with ease.

Remember, if you don't understand an exercise term, just ask!

Workout Ideas

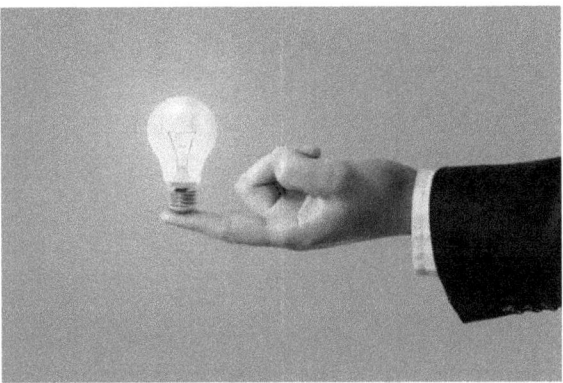

There are plenty of different workout options to help ease your way into fitness, ones that are fun and get results fast.

All you've gotta do, is open your mind to all the different options. Don't be afraid to try something new, to figure out what marries best with you.

A few of the essentials in a complete body workout are:

*Stretching
*Aerobic activity
*Strength training

Livestrong says, your physical fitness is the ability of your circulatory, muscular, and respiratory systems to handle elevated demands of intensity, where you have the staying power to perform daily tasks, without tiring, while reducing the risk of injury or sickness.

STRETCHING

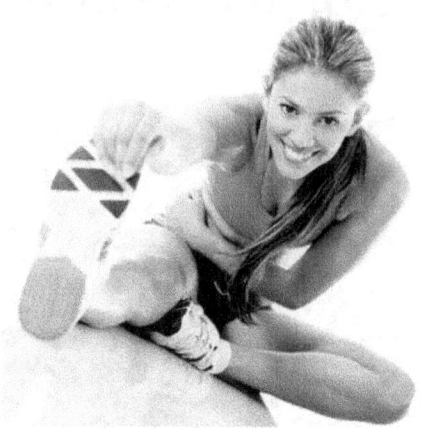

I likely sound like a recorder, but it's vital you stretch before and after your workout, and even during if possible. Having your muscles loose, ready and able to perform, helps you steer clear of serious injury.

Here are a few of the basic stretches:

Calf Stretch

Your calf muscle runs along the bottom half of the back of your leg. Very important for running, jumping, and even walking. To stretch your calf muscle, face the wall and place your hands against the wall in a pushup position, while lunging your left knee forward with your right leg extended back behind you, with both toes pointed forward. The idea is to gently straighten your back leg, while leaning forward.

Don't bounce or over stretch.

Hold each stretch for about thirty seconds. Alternate legs two or three times.

Side Stretch

Stand sideways beside a wall. Cross your legs, and place your left hand on the wall for support, while you extend your right arm sideways over your head towards the wall. You should feel the stretch up your side.

Hold this stretch for about thirty seconds.

Repeat with the other side, and complete two or three times.

Quad Stretch

Stand beside a chair for balance, upright with your hips square. With your right arm, pull your right leg behind you up towards your buttocks. Make sure you don't lean forward.

Pull your foot towards your buttocks until you feel a nice stretch.

Hold it for thirty seconds and repeat with other leg. Stretch each quad two or three times.

Hip Stretch

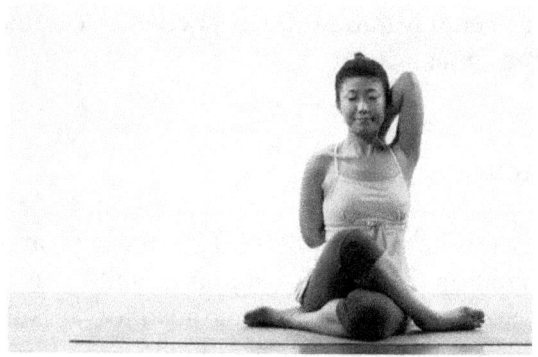

Sit down with knees bent. Cross your right leg over the left. Twist your body to the right. Place your left elbow to your right knee, while twisting to the right.

You should feel a gentle pull along your right side. Hold it for thirty seconds and alternate.

Repeat two or three times each side.

Hamstring Stretch

Lie down on your back with your feet close to a wall. Put your left heel against the wall, raise your right leg straight in the air, and gently straighten until you feel a stretch along the back of your leg.

Hold for thirty seconds, alternate, and repeat two or three times.

Back/Shoulder Stretch

Stand with feet shoulder width apart. Clasp your hands together behind your back, bend forward at the waist, and try and raise your clasped hands up towards the ceiling.

You should feel a nice stretch in your back and shoulders.

Hold for thirty seconds and repeat two or three times.

Head/Neck Stretch

Stand with feet shoulder width apart. With your eyes facing forward, tilt your right ear down toward your right shoulder. You'll feel the stretch along the left side of your neck.

Alternate sides, and hold each stretch for thirty seconds.

Repeat two or three times each side.

Knee/Chest Stretch for Lower Back

Lay on your back and bring your right knee up towards your chest, while your left leg stays straight. Clasp your arms around your leg and pull in towards chest.

You'll feel this gentle stretch in your lower back. Hold thirty seconds, alternate, and repeat two or three times.

Cat Stretch

This stretch will help loosen you up. Triggering blood flow to your back, shoulders, and core area.

Get down on all fours. Arch your back up towards the ceiling like a cat, while hunching your shoulders over, and pushing your head toward the floor.

Hold for thirty seconds.

Then lift your head up, pull your shoulders back, and push your midsection towards the floor, while sticking your buttocks out.

Hold thirty seconds. Repeat both stretches two or three times.

Triceps Stretch

Put your right palm between your shoulder blades on your back. Make sure your elbow is pointing towards the ceiling.

With your left hand, slowly pull your elbow towards your head, using your left hand.

Hold for thirty seconds.

Do the same with the other side. Repeat two or three times each side.

Biceps Stretch

Stand perpendicular to a wall at the end of it. With your right arm facing the wall, stand almost an arm's length away, and rest the fingertips of your right hand on the end of the wall.

Twist your upper body gently to the left with your fingers still on the end on the wall, pushing your shoulder forward to feel a stretch in in your upper arm.

Hold for thirty seconds.

Alternate arms, and repeat sequence two or three times.

Lunges

These will help stretch your legs. Stand with feet together. Lunge forward with your right knee, keeping your right leg straight behind you. Don't go past 90 degrees, or you're overextending.

Just lunge far enough forward to feel a gentle stretch. Hold for thirty seconds.

Repeat with other leg, and complete ten with each. Do two or three sets.

Stretching is something that'll help prevent injury, gain mobility and agility, along with improving balance and coordination. There are lots of beginner stretching programs online to choose from.

Or you can set one up with your personal trainer, if that's the route you choose.

AEROBIC/CARDIOVASCULAR ACTIVITY

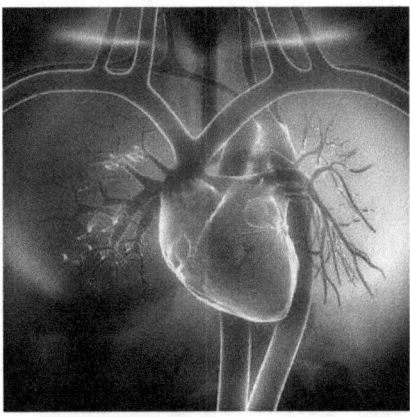

Improving your fitness level requires intense aerobic conditioning, getting your heart rate pumping, and blood flowing masterfully throughout your body, transporting increased oxygen, vitamins, and minerals, to your major organs and supporting systems, so you can exercise longer and harder.

Experts suggest at least thirty minutes a day of cardiovascular activity, with forty-five minutes being ideal.

What's important, is you think carefully before deciding on your aerobic activities. Set yourself up for success. Figure out what you enjoy.

If you really loathe the thought of committing to the gym and walking or running on the treadmill, then don't do it.

Instead, join a walking or biking group to start!

If you work better with other people around as support and motivation, then make certain that's exactly what you do. If you're not a self-motivator, don't try and train solo.

It's also critical to note, you should rotate your cardio activity each day. Three times a week you might do an aerobics session for beginners. The other days, use the stepper or cross trainer at the gym, or go for a brisk walk.

Diversity is very important. It'll starve off boredom, and help maximum results, by keeping your mind thinking, and body working different groups of muscles, simultaneously. OD'ing on routine, in fitness for beginners, will take the wind out of your sails.

If you tend to veer off course in life, you'll want to hire a personal training to set you up and keep on your case.

Definitely something to think about, and worth every penny in my opinion.

Getting into great cardiovascular shape gives you more energy, optimism, improved metabolism, less toxic buildup, better internal system efficiency, and so much more.

Bottom line is, your body was custom designed for physical challenge daily, whether you like it or not. Cardiovascular activity on a routine basis, is a large part of it.

One other point: Walking around the block without effort at a snail's pace **DOES NOT COUNT** as cardio activity, nor does biking slower than a turtle. *SOME* effort is required!

You should be working up a sweat. Do it like you mean it, instead of whining, complaining, and making lame excuses.

CHALLENGE yourself so it counts!

Here are a few great options for aerobic exercise:

*Biking
*Brisk Walking/Jogging/Running
*Swimming
*Hiking
*Gardening (fast pace)
*Aerobics Classes
*Boot Camps
*Treadmill
*Stair Climber
*Cross Trainer
*Elliptical Trainer
*Water Sports
*Soccer

*Basketball/Volleyball/Tennis/Hockey/Ringette
*Gymnastics/Cheerleading
*Yoga (specific types)
*Skipping
*Skating
*Martial Arts
*Cross Country Skiing
*Tobogganing
*Cross Fit

This gives you a medley of activities to choose from, to get your heart rate into *cardio workout* zone. Your backup thinking can be, that picking up the pace with yard and housework, also constitutes a workout, if you breathe heavy long enough!

And don't even think of cheating, unless you like cheating yourself.

P.S. Sex counts, when you're in the driver's seat!

STRENGTH TRAINING

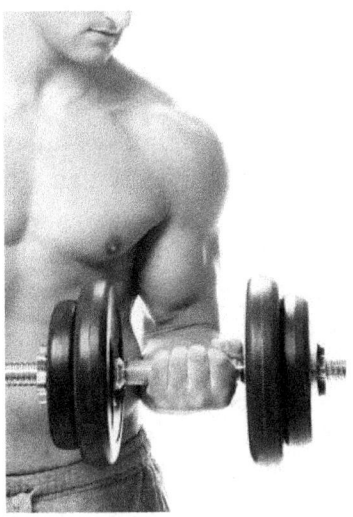

Complete full body workouts need strength training. Whether you're working with free weights, weight machines, or resistance training, having sexy strong muscles is absolute in overall good health.

Strength training empowers you to look like a million bucks, and feel good like a zillion, challenging physical exercise that zones into using resistance, to force your muscles to contract, build strength, and improve body function as a whole.

Figuring out what strength training maneuvers fox trot nicely with your personal goals and strategies, is your first wise-owl move.

There are oodles of options to build your muscles strong. If you have a job requiring lots of physical effort, this count this towards your strength training goals.

For example, farmers get plenty of muscle building every day working on the farm. From lifting hay bales and bags of feed, to moving heavy parts to fix machinery, and lifting baby animals into their pens.

If you happen to run across a farmer somewhere, ask to check out their pipes. I guarantee you're gonna get wowed!

If you work in a factory that requires sorting and lifting heavy objects all day, that counts too! Just make sure you're bending at the knees and NOT the back!

Lifting weights is popular for muscle building. You can choose to use weights or machines to start, where experts point out combination is best. Don't forget diversity is queen. It starves off boredom, maximizes calories burned, speeds up the weight loss process, and gets you to goals faster.

We're going to focus on weight training, and break it down into upper body, lower body, and core. A little of each to start is a cool move, simply because you won't be lifting heavy weights, or very many sets with each exercise.

CIP (Cathy's Important Point) - Weight training is something you need to ease yourself into, to avoid injury, or learning the wrong form/technique. Using incorrect techniques, warrants most of your training useless.

According to *Healthy Living*, using proper form throughout an exercise, makes the appropriate muscles work harder, triggering faster results.

After you get used to weight training in general, you should transition into upper body one day, lower body another, and core for the third day, with at least a day's rest in between different muscle groups.

Upper Body

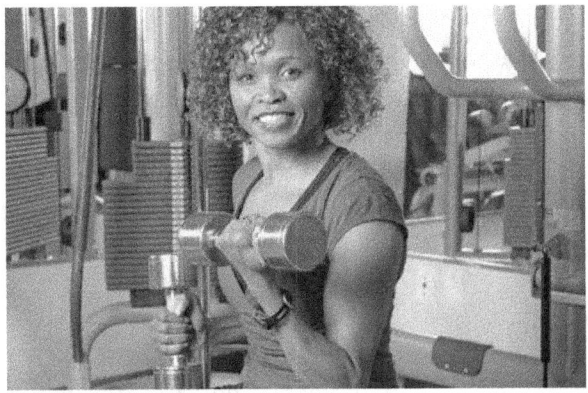

Bench Press

Lay down on the bench with a light dumbbell in each hand.

CIP - You aren't trying to win a weight lifting competition. You want to focus on great form. This requires very light weights to start. So you can get used to the motion.

With your head looking straight at the ceiling, and your knees bent comfortably and set on the bench, you're going to push the dumbbells up slowly and controlled towards the ceiling, while breathing out.

Do this for a three count. Pause, and lower back down while breathing in, to a two count.

Repeat this ten times, rest a minute, and do two more sets.

Biceps

Stand feet shoulder width apart with a dumbbell in each hand. Your palms should be facing away from you. In a controlled fashion, curl your left arm up towards your chest, while keeping your elbow tight into your body.

Make sure it's perpendicular to the ground, so it's just the top half of your arm moving upwards. Move up for a three count, and down for a two count.

Do ten reps with each arm, rest, and repeat two more sets each arm.

Triceps

This muscle is along the back top half of your arm. Stand bent over 90 degrees at the waist, with a weight in your right hand. Supporting yourself with your left hand on the bench or a chair, bend your right elbow up, keeping it parallel to the floor.

Extend the weight backwards towards the height of your elbow, to a straightened position. Be sure to extend the weight upwards, making your arm straight. Don't drop your arm down. While keeping your back flat and head forward.

Repeat ten reps, pause, and do two more sets of ten. Alternate arms.

Shoulder Press

Stand with your feet shoulder width apart, knees slightly bent, and weights resting on your shoulders. Push the weights upwards towards the ceiling up over your head, until arms are extended. Then slowly lower back down to starting position.

Repeat this ten times, pause, and do two more sets.

*This can also be done effectively with a shoulder press machine.

Pulldown

Sit down on the machine and grasp the bar. Pull the bar down in a slow and controlled motion towards your shoulders. Pause at the bottom, and slowly raise the bar back up to the starting position.

Repeat this ten times, pause, and do two more sets.

*Be sure to keep your back straight, and shoulders back.

Shoulder Fly

Sit on the machine, grasp the handles, and let the pads rest on the top of your arms. Slowly raise your arms up so your forearms are parallel to the ground. Then lower back down to the standard three count.

Repeat ten times, pause, and do two more sets.

Lower Body

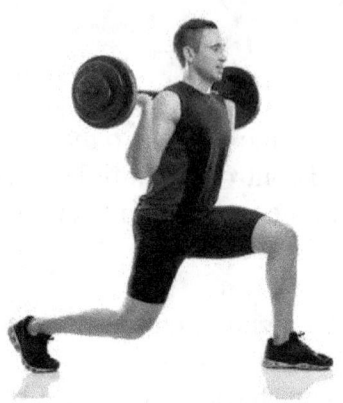

I would like to mention, most cardio exercises work your lower body a lot. So you don't really need as much of a focus to start, with lower body weights. This doesn't mean you can ignore it. But if you only get two or three different lower body strength training exercises in per session, you don't need to cry.

Lower body training should happen 1-2 times a week.

Squats

I can't stress how fantabulous squats are for working your lower body. Toning and strengthening your core, legs, and buttocks. I LOVE feeling it in my butt the day after!

CIP - Proper technique is EVERYTHING in a squat!

*Keep your back flat
*Cute butt sticking out
*Eyes forward
*Head straight
*Shoulders back

Stand with your feet shoulder width apart, and a light bar across your shoulders, at least until you're used to the motion.

Keeping your back straight and butt sticking out, slowly lower yourself down to a 90 degree angle to a three count, and back up again. This counts as one rep.

Repeat this ten times, pause, and do two more sets. You should feel your thighs burning when finished.

Extensions

Sit on the machine with legs hooked snuggly underneath the pads. Slowly extend your legs up to a straightened position, and then back down to the starting position.

Repeat this ten times, pause, and then do two more sets.

*You're going to find some exercises you love, and others you hate. I happen to have a love-hate relationship with extensions. I detest doing them, but love the results!

Hamstrings

Sit on the machine and place your legs on top of the pads. Slowly use your muscles to lower your legs down towards your buttocks. Then back up to the starting position in a slow and controlled three count fashion.

Complete ten reps, take a break, and do two more sets.

Core

There are literally hundreds of different core exercises. We're going to look at a few to get you started. This core muscle group is actually known as your rectus abdominus, close to the surface of the skin.

The five core muscles are:

Rectus Abdominus - The most popular abs muscle. It runs from the bottom of your ribs, to the top of your pelvis.

Obliques - These are found on your sides and lower back. The three types are transverse, internal, and external.

Erector Spinae - These are the eight muscles that run up both sides of your spine. They run from the base of your skull to base of the sacrum.

Transverse Abdominus - This is the thin wide muscle that runs around your abdominal cavity.

Quadratus Lumborum - A deep muscle running from the bottom of your ribs, to the top of your pelvis.

Note: After you become skilled in ab work, you can challenge yourself by placing a weight on your tummy while executing your exercises! Talk about a killer workout!

Simple Crunch

The crunch targets the middle area of your abdominals, around your navel. Simply lie on your back with bent knees. Hands clasped behind your head. Slowly pull your chest towards your knees in a crunched position using your abdominals, slightly lifting your shoulders off the ground. You don't need a big motion to feel this one.

Slowly lower yourself back down to the starting position.

Complete this ten times, rest, then do another two sets.

*Make sure you keep your abdominals contracted start to finish, for maximum effectiveness.

Pelvic Tilt

These are great cuz you can do the anywhere.

Lay on your back with feet flat on the floor, and knees bent. Place your arms outstretched to your sides, in line with shoulders.

Breathe out and push your hips toward the ceiling, squeezing your butt at the top. Then slowly lower yourself back down, without resting or touching the ground with your butt.

Repeat ten times in a slow and controlled motion, pause, and do two more sets.

Obliques

These core muscles help to bend your torso and rotate it. Lie on your back with your feet flat and knees slightly bent. Lift your legs off the ground, twist to the right, and lower them, but don't touch the ground.

Ensure your arms are extended out to your sides and flat on the ground, along with your shoulders.

Bring the legs back up to the starting point, and rotate to the other side.

Repeat this sequence five times on each side, rest, and repeat one more time.

Lower Abdominals

Lie on your back with knees slightly bent, arms to your sides. Put your feet straight up in the air to start, lowering them slowly down towards the ground until the touch slightly.

Bring your legs back to their starting position and repeat ten times.

Make sure your motion is slow and controlled, and bring your legs down to the count of three.

Do two more sets.

Plank

This is excellent for all your core muscles. Lay face down on the ground. Lift yourself up off the ground, supporting yourself with your forearms. So, up on your elbows if you will. Ensure your body stays straight, and your core muscles are keeping your back flat and in line with the rest of your body, right down to your toes.

This is called the plank position.

Hold this position firm for ten seconds to start.

Repeat this three times with a thirty second rest in between.

As you get stronger, lengthen the plank time by ten second intervals. This should be challenging for you. If it isn't, you need to increase the duration.

Fitness Alert - You've got to start somewhere right? If you can only do a walk around the block a couple times, then that's where you start from. As long as you're slowly improving, putting in the effort to build your cardiovascular capacity, then you're moving forward.

Before you know it, you'll be walking at a brisk pace for thirty minutes!

It's all about progress, and setting yourself up for success with REASONABLE expectations. The number one reason beginners fail in fitness, is because they expect the impossible. Slow and steady wins the race here. Always push yourself gently to do more, and you'll reach your goals - believe it!

My Thoughts . . .
Stretching is probably the most important aspect of getting fit. If you don't stretch regularly, you're going to injure yourself, which doesn't help your fitness goals

I'm a little bit different here, because cardio is my favorite part of working out. It's where I get to get my heart rate working overtime, release my stress, and re-energize myself, by tapping into my infinite endorphin stores.

I can't tell you what the best cardio activity is for you. I don't know if you have any health conditions, if you're claustrophobic, or if out with nature is the only route to go for you.

So it's up to you to try out different activities, even ones you "think" you won't ever enjoy, and figure out what works for you. Aerobic conditioning can be fun and effective if you want it to be.

Of course, strength training to build muscle is also very important, if you want to get strong, kiss fat goodbye, and keep it off by boosting your metabolism. Lifting weights for just fifteen minutes, three days a week, is really all you need.

Equipment to Purchase

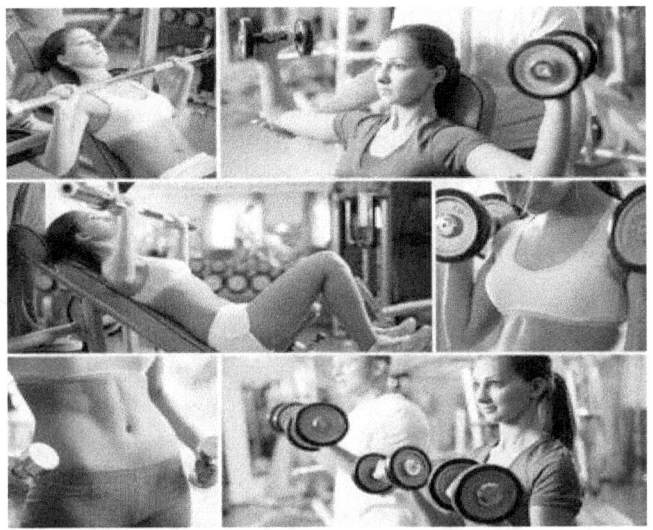

Particularly if you're pinched for time, it makes sense to buy a few pieces of gym equipment.

This eliminates excuses for not working out! Including the just plain lazy-butt one!

And this move is even better if you're naturally self-motivated and have a scary busy schedule.

FACT: You don't need to spend an arm and a leg on equipment to get started.

Garage sales are a fantabulous place to get cardio equipment and weights dirt cheap. There's also the newspaper, and postings at local gyms. Lucky for you, oodles of wanna-be-fit people buy crazy expensive equipment, and never use it.

All you need is a piece of cardio equipment, and either some free weights, or a strength training device. Exercise balls and bands also work well. Universal gyms are awesome too. And buying used, or even taking it off the hands of a neighbor, is definitely an option.

Have a look around, and figure out what suits your lifestyle best.

Here are a few pieces of equipment that are popular in a home. First, we'll look at cardio equipment, then strength training, stretching, and other.

CARDIO EQUIPMENT FOR HOME

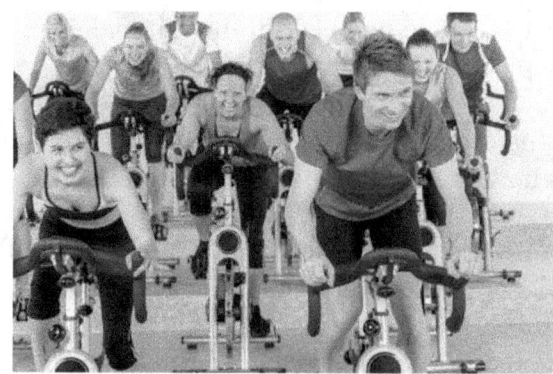

Treadmills

Good treadmills can be very expensive and really heavy. If you buy a cheap light one, I'm telling you now, it'll be a waste of money. They don't usually perform very well. Cheaper isn't better with a treadmill.

Before buying, make sure you at least talk with a cardio expert from a sports equipment store. Combine that with the information you've got, and some internet investigation, and you're equipped to get a great piece of cardio equipment, within your budget.

*Of course there's always your legs! Walking, jogging, running, and hiking, are all fantastic ways to get your heart rate up. And the best thing is, you don't need anything but a quality pair of runners.

Fitness Alert - It's critical that you wear good quality shoes on your feet at all times. All sorts of health issues can arise from improper footwear. From simple blisters and calluses, to issues with your bones, muscles, and tendons, from wearing shoes that either don't fit, or have the support your body requires. You're on your feet all the time. The least you can do is wear comfortable footwear that supports and fits your foot properly.

Ellipticals

This is a fantastic piece of cardio equipment that works both your upper and lower body simultaneously. A key advantage is minute wear and tear on your joints.

Nothing like running does for instance.

It's a cushioned motion, that gives your heart a great workout. On the flip side, some people find the motion takes a few tries to get used to, because it takes some coordination. No worries though, you'll eventually get it!

Having a piece of equipment like this in your home is pricey. A good quality one is at least $1500. If you can afford it, and are gonna use it, then go for it!

Don't go with a light one, and make sure you test it out first. This is one piece of equipment you don't want to muck up on.

It's best to speak with a fitness equipment expert before buying. I will say, this is one of my favorite pieces. Although first prize for me goes to the spin bike, which is next.

Bikes

A very popular piece of equipment indeed. Most people can get their cardio on a stationary bike. Even people with bad knees and hips. More pluses are, stationary bikes aren't very pricy, and garage sales often feature them.

BONUS - They're safer than regular cycling. If you have mobility or balance issues for example, a stationary bike is an excellent option for cardio.

I prefer a spin bike myself. They are stationary bikes meant for hard riding, standing up on, and moving around. These bikes are used specifically in spin classes, which you've likely seen at the gym before.

Other than boot camps, I believe this is the toughest cardio workout you can get. And the beauty of it, is you control the pace. I love it fast and hard, so it works for me.

Stair Climbers/Stepper

The steppers pretty popular in the gym. Recently, prices have come down. But you'll still need to opt for the higher end steppers and stair climbers, if you don't want to waste money. The better models are heavier and well worth it. But you'll have to figure out your budget first, and which models you prefer.

Climbers work your lower body really well, tightening your buttocks nicely, and toning your thigh area. This is a great piece of cardio equipment to start out with. You can pick your pace and intensity level, and work your way up.

Years ago I had a pretty light hydraulic one I got for a hundred bucks. It wasn't the best, but it did the trick for the days I didn't make it to the gym.

Rowing

Rowers are another awesome way to get your cardio. They work both upper and lower body effectively, and help with stretching, flexibility, and mobility. The resistance and pace is set by you, so you can start slow and work your way up. Rowing machines are fairly affordable, which means you can get a good quality model without breaking the bank. This is the piece of equipment rowers in training often use off season.

You should be able to grab a decent one for around two hundred dollars.

Skipping

All you need here, is a skipping rope and a desire to get sweaty. Skipping is an incredibly tough workout that takes time to master. If you can start doing 5 minutes, you're in great shape.

A skipping rope is nice on the wallet, cuz all you need are your runners, a skipping rope, and very little space. An excellent choice for traveling too, when you're camping out in hotel rooms.

Aerobics

Many people that are self-motivated, and use aerobic videos to get a great cardio workout in. There are so many to choose from; kickboxing, hip-hop dance, and high-energy cardio. It's important you get at least a couple different tapes if this is your route. Mixing things up starves off boredom for one.

No matter your level in introductory fitness, challenge yourself!

Don't be afraid to combine two or three of the cardio activities. Maybe get one good piece of equipment, like a treadmill or stationary bike, and compliment it with a skipping rope, and maybe a few aerobics tapes.

Get your body sweating, have fun, and keep it diversified and exciting.

STRENGTH TRAINING EQUIPMENT

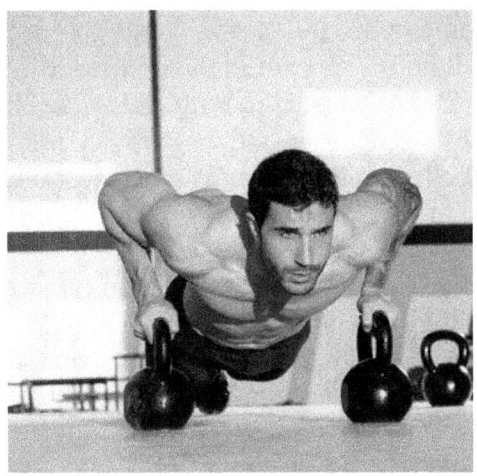

There are a whole whack of fantastic pieces of muscle building equipment, depending on your budget. You can spend very little, or oodles, and build your body sexy strong.

Dumbbells

These are something everyone should have at home, even when training elsewhere. With a few dumbbells, you can work every muscle on your body.

Starting off slow with the basic muscle building exercises for your upper and lower body. Then working your way up in variety, tempo, pace, and rhythm. Each of these factors will positively impact your muscles, body, and overall workout.

Dumbbells are cheap, and take up next to no room. You can even take them with you when you travel. Just fifteen minutes, three days a week, is all you need to start building.

Home Gyms

Universal home gyms are another great choice, giving your muscles a full body workout in the comfort of your home. Some gyms use resistance, and others have weights.

Both are effective, and you've just gotta test them out and figure out what works for you.

The price range goes from affordable, to crazy expensive, depending on your wants, needs, and budget. If you enjoy working out at the gym, but can't cuz of your schedule or some other circumstance, a home gym may be perfect for you.

They do take up a little bit of space, depending on the size you want. But are definitely well worth it. To me, it's diversity at your fingertips.

Resistance Bands

This is another great piece of equipment that's cheap, and takes up no space. These bands usually come with sample exercises, and can be used safely for building muscle while stretching. Also fantabulous for improving flexibility and mobility, so I'll mention them again when we get to that section.

Bands are versatile. You can shorten them for more resistance if you like, challenging your muscles. It's smart to start off with little resistance, to make sure your form is correct. Then you can kick it up a notch or two, and start challenging yourself more.

Medicine Ball

This is great for building muscle and cardio simultaneously. Depending on the weight of the ball, you can do exercises to build muscle, or just make your cardio activity harder. Medicine balls don't cost a lot, and it doesn't hurt to have them around to help change things up, or just work a little harder.

For example, if you're executing squats, and getting pretty comfortable with them, adding a medicine ball will challenge your muscle strength and lung capacity.

Shocking your system is a wonderful thing!

Fitness Alert - Technique is everything when you're getting your body fit. If you perform an exercise incorrectly, you'll injure yourself, or it won't be very effective. Putting in the effort and not getting results sucks!

It's frustrating, and one of the main reasons people quit training, according to Men's Health.

Make sure you're doing the exercises correctly, and if you aren't sure, just ask someone who's qualified. You can't afford not to.

You don't have to lift oodles of weight to build beautiful lean muscle. Weight lifting helps you look leaner and lose weight faster, because muscle burns more calories than fat does, actually boosting your metabolism.

Even when you're taking a nap, you're burning more calories than if you weren't lifting weights. A measly fifteen minutes, about three times a week, is all you need to start.

Don't think about it, just do it!

STRETCHING AND OTHER

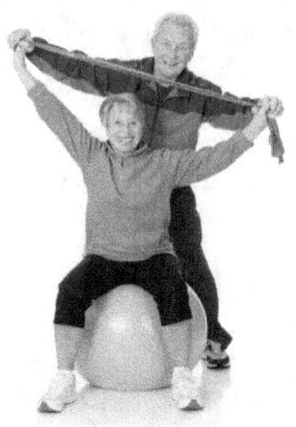

We're going to talk about stretching equipment, and any other pieces you might like when exercising for beginners. Remember, there are lots and lots of different stretching devices out there, and you need to experiment a little to figure out what compliments your preferences and tolerances.

To start, you just need your body, the knowledge, and the desire to get stretching. But if you'd like some equipment to motivate you or assist you, there's always:

Resistance Bands

Yes, we mentioned bands already for strength training. But resistance bands are excellent for stretching too. They'll assist you in completing stretches you might not be flexible enough to do right now otherwise.
For example, there's a stretch behind the back, where you try and reach your hands together. Most people can't touch their hands. But using a resistance band, gives you the stretch you want, and gets you closer to actually grabbing your hands.

Resistance bands also help you with form, and give you a touch of resistance when stretching, which builds you stronger.

Mat

This isn't a must, but having a nice mat to stretch and weight train on, is a luxury item that's affordable! It's good for your head too, because it signals that it's time to get down to business, to focus on your training.

Of course, you can always use a towel on your floor. That works too!

Cruncher

There are all sorts of ab machines out there, ranging in price. A flag of caution, is try before you buy.

More often than not, you'll find a diverse range of core exercises without equipment, does the trick to start. And when you get advanced, you can incorporate dumbbells into your ab routine. I love doing that.

Don't be afraid to experiment a little, but always start off slow.

Exercise Ball

An exercise ball is great for using with weights, core, and stretching. It adds diversity in your routine, and challenges you to push it to the next level. An exercise ball is great for form, and supports your neck and back well for core and strength training exercises.

An exercise ball has a zillion uses. A fantistico piece of equipment for you!

Actual Stretching Machines

There are actually stretching machines that assist with stretching. Take heed, they're very pricey! I wouldn't opt for one. If you're stretching properly, you don't need one.

Maybe when you're experienced, you'll find a piece of stretching equipment that's helpful for a specific purpose.

I just wouldn't go investing right now.

Weight Belt

Should you or shouldn't you? A weight belt can actually get you into a whole whack of trouble injury-wise. It makes you believe you have a stronger back, which makes you lazy in form.

If you're form's crappy, you'll injure yourself. So unless you are recovering from a back injury, and understand the belt is just giving you a little more stability, I would steer clear of it.

I'm sure you see some macho men strutting their stuff in the gym with their gynormous weight belt on. Chances are pretty good they're not even wearing the right size.

Just be smart here, please. It's more of a statement than functional.

Ankle/Wrist Weights

You may or may not need these right away. But ankle or wrist weights are an awesome way to challenge yourself a little more. If you're wearing them when power walking for instance, this will take your cardio workout up a few notches.

Wrist weight are great for strength training too. Just to give you a little extra. They take up little space and are budget friendly. Great to have around just in case!

There are all sorts of tools you can use to help you get your body fit. It's up to you to decide how much you are looking to invest, and what your preferences and tolerances are. It kills me to see people unload lots of money on equipment that either lets them down, or they never really intended to use anyway.

Just be smart in your choices. Buy only what you need. Test everything before you write the cheque. And make sure you've got a plan to use it.

You not going to lose fat, build muscle, and increase your flexibility, mobility, and motility, if your exercise equipment is dusty!

Final Thoughts

I'm not going to sugar coat anything. Getting fit isn't easy, but that doesn't mean it can't be meaningful and fun. It may take some time for exercising to grow on you. So if you really don't "feel" like exercising for the first few weeks, that's okay. But you're going to do it anyway.

Treat it like a job, and don't think about it so much. Just do it.

In time, you'll figure out what exercise routine works for you, your preferences, tolerances, and limitations. Set your goals to challenge your limitations. Understanding any sort of exercise is good for your mind, body, and soul.

Exercise builds strength and clearer thinking, triggers positivity, and decreases those pesky aches and pains you've accepted as normal.

It's time to slip on your good quality runners, and take the first step to bigger and better in everything. Create your plan and execute!

Last Thoughts…

*THANK-YOU for reading my masterpiece. I hope you learned a little something, or at least got a few smiles.
*I would appreciate a millisecond or three of your time for a quick review, to help me build my masterful book empire higher.
*Whatever you do, don't forget to smile, and of course, check out my website for more of my e-Book masterpieces at: flawlesscreativewriting.com

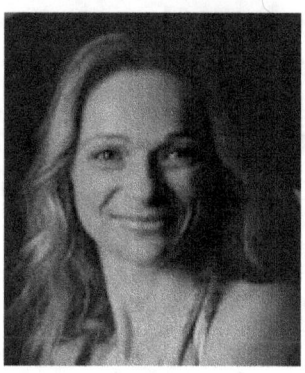

Cathy☺

www.ingramcontent.com/pod-product-compliance
Lightning Source LLC
Chambersburg PA
CBHW070603290526
45790CB00002B/760